DUKAN DIET

How To Lose Weight Quickly Using The Dukan Diet Plan
In 30 Days Or Less Is The Ultimate Guide To The Dukan
Diet

*(How To Commence With The Attack Phase Of The Dukan
Diet)*

I0083586

Germain Deschenes

TABLE OF CONTENT

Chapter 1: Diet During The Phase Of Consolidation

The third phase of the Dukan Diet is the consolidation phase, which is characterized by a minor relaxation of the meal plan so that Decanals can enjoy wine once or twice per week, but only if they consume a large amount of protein the following day.

Lean Green Protein Smoothie: The first item on our schedule is the lean green protein smoothie. The beverage can also be consumed during the Vegetable plus protein phase of the Cruise Phase, but not during the protein-only phase. Ingredients include 2 2 celery stalk, 2 cup of cold water, 2 teaspoon of flax seed oil, 2 cup of frozen spinach, 2 cup of kale, and 2 tablespoon of vanilla protein powder. This recipe takes approximately 2 0 minutes to prepare and yields two servings per day. All of

1

these ingredients are added to a blender and processed until homogeneous.

Spaghetti Squash: The spaghetti squash recipe can be used in both the consolidation phase and the stabilization phase, which is the final phase of the Dukan diet cycle. It is also suitable for the vegetable and protein phase of the cruise cycle. This recipe is easily prepared by poking a hole in the spaghetti squash and cooking the spaghetti for 8 -10 minutes per pound in the oven. Allow the spaghetti to settle for a set amount of time before proceeding. Now, open the linguine and remove any seeds that may be present. Now you can add salt, pepper, or any other flavoring ingredient you desire.

Chicken and Pumpkin: A very elegant, attractive, and straightforward recipe. You may consume a high-protein diet of chicken and vegetables to meet your protein requirements for this cycle. The most important ingredients for this dish are chicken breast, mushrooms, pumpkins, onions, parsley, light milk, salt, and pepper. The flesh is first cut to the required size before being seared on both sides. Next, minced onions and mushrooms are added. Add salt and pepper and continue cooking for a while. Now divide the meat, onion, and mushroom.Add pumpkin to the sauce, then position the meat on top. Now pour milk on top of it.Cook it for some time before serving it.

⬜ Onion and Pepper Salad: The ideal combination of chilly and heat.The recipe is founded on the well-known fact that salads are a person's primary source of protein. Although the preparation time for the recipe is approximately 2 2.10 hours, once the recipe has been prepared, it can be consumed five times per day, which is the quantity recommended by the protein chart. The primary ingredients are bay leaf, vinegar, salt, pepper, onions, bell pepper, and a small amount of sugar.The vegetable is first salted and allowed to sit overnight.Afterwards, eliminate any excess liquid using a sieve. Now prepare the marinade by boiling 10

00 ml of water, Vinegar Sweetener, bay leaf, and all spices.Add the vegetables and simmer them for five minutes.Immediately pour the vegetable and liquid into the receptacle.Place the canister upside down on a towel to dry.The container is then stored in a cabinet for a very long time.Once opened, the beverage is refrigerated.Add cheese or another ingredient, and the product is available for consumption.

2.8) Dukan Diet Throughout the Stability Phase

The fourth and final phase of the Dukan diet is the final stroke you must take to overcome the Obesity Problem and become the person with a charming personality you've always desired to be. This phase offers a permanent reprieve from the obesity threat if four principles are followed beforehand;

2 -Have consumed whatever you desire, but the diet must have contained an unlimited amount of protein and vegetables in previous phases.

2-Have devoted at least one day per week to consuming only protein.

Minimum of three liters of water per day.

8 -Have adequately moved your body in the previous three phases and continue to do so.

Also included in this phase are recipes designed specifically to satisfy the daily needs of this plan's user.

Light Bacon Omelette: Incorporate this omelette into your daily regimen.With a preparation time of only 10 minutes and a boiling time of 10 to 2 0 minutes, the omelette is simple to prepare at any time. The essential ingredients are Fat-Reduced Bacon, 8 Fresh eggs, an Appropriate Quantity of Skim Milk (one with very little fat), Garlic, and Black Pepper. The first step in the procedure is to cut the bacon into thin segments. Combine all of the ingredients in a jar or receptacle, and then sprinkle them with pepper. They are heated in a griddle.Avoid using oil whenever feasible. Cook the omelette until it is done. Serve promptly.

Salmon Burger: The salmon burger is an excellent recipe for fast food lovers who have been famished since the beginning of this diet. The dish can be served once after 2 0 minutes of preparation and 8 minutes of heating. The primary components include oat bran, egg, mustard, fat-free quark, and cured salmon. Owen. For preparation, combine all the ingredients in a small basin, and then microwave for a few minutes.Make bread segments and spread mustard on the bread. Make a burger with the second portion of bread.

▢ Chicken Korma: Specifically created for the subcontinental population. The poultry korma provides a high amount of protein to its consumer.The dish can be consumed four times per day. The cooking time is only 6 0 minutes and the preparatory time is only 20 minutes.

Onions, fat-free quark, mustard, garam masala, chicken breast, and lemon juice are the ingredients in this dish.For its preparation, create an onion paste. Mustard and Quark. Add garam masala to it. Now, cut the chicken into desired segments and add it to the bowl so that it is completely coated with paste.Leave for some time in refrigeration. Alternatively, preheat the oven. Now place the chicken in the oven dish and heat for approximately 6 0 minutes at 200C.Serve the dish while it is still steaming and add lemon to enhance the flavor.

Three of the Best Smoothie Recipes

Enough with the recipes already! It's time to indulge in something delectable. We are aware that no one can survive without daily sugar consumption, as it is an absolute necessity. Shakes and smoothies play a crucial role in this regard, as they provide the essential hydration and protein content as well as the variety of flavor that everyone seeks. Here are some recipes for smoothies.

⬚   Banana and Strawberry Smoothie: The Strawberry banana smoothie combines the flavorful strawberry flavor with the protein-rich banana. Optimized for optimal nutritional content, the smoothie can easily satisfy your daily protein and carbohydrate needs.If someone wishes to enhance the protein content, protein powder can be added to maximize the daily protein intake. Banana, skim milk, vanilla extract, artificial sweetener, and a few ice crystals comprise the majority of the ingredients. To prepare the recipe, place all the ingredients in a blender and combine until a smooth mixture is obtained. It contains only about 0.7 grams of fat.

Mango-banana-pineapple smoothie: The next item on our list is the mango-banana-pineapple smoothie. We explicitly mention this smoothie recipe because many people around the world have mango or banana as their preferred fruit. These two items with additional pineapple flavor leave a residue in the mouth that is difficult to eliminate.With only 2 .6 grams of total fat and 20 grams of protein, this recipe can be consumed four times a day at any time. It pairs especially well with breakfast and keeps the Dieter energized throughout the day. The primary components are 2 ounce each of vanilla, skim milk, mango, pineapple, and banana.Blend all ingredients in a blender, then serve to visitors. You will get a positive response for sure.

Mocha Banana Smoothie: The Mocha banana Smoothie is third on our list. Smoothies, renowned for their unique flavor, are primarily consumed in Africa and neighboring regions. The lipid content is limited to 0.9g, while the protein content is 10 .8 g.The primary components are condensed milk, vanilla, coffee crystals, cocoa powder, bananas, and sugar. Simply purée them for 10 to

2 0 minutes and consume a minimum of 2 servings per day.

Tropical Avocado Smoothie: despite its color, the finest smoothie is the tropical avocado smoothie.Smoothies are most popular in tropical regions, where they have been consumed as a daily beverage for centuries. The primary constituents consist of coconut, avocado, fresh ginger, vanilla, lime juice, and a few other conventional foods. Simply blend the mixture for five to ten minutes to obtain the finest tropical flavor.

Strawberry Almond milk Smoothie: The last item on our list is a fresh strawberry and yogurt smoothie that can be consumed twice daily. The primary constituents are yogurt, strawberry, sugar-free almond milk, and low-fat yogurt. Blend them together, and you're done. This smoothie may provide you with the finest smoothie experience you've ever had.

8 - The Seven Day Dukan Diet Plan

Stop donning clothes that do not match your personality, with your stomach protruding from your shirt and pants. Today is the day of decision-making. Today is the beginning of your finest nutritional diet, "The Dukan Seven-Day Meal Plan."

This diet begins with pure protein and gradually adds other components such as vegetables, lipids, and starchy foods, etc., so that you can achieve a balanced diet over the course of seven days. This plan also emphasizes increasing daily activity, whether through exercise or simple walking, so that the dieter's metabolic rate increases over time.

Day 2 of the Diet Plan: The day is a pure protein day, as it is part of the first attack phase, so the various protein recipes listed above can be consumed in excess.

The second day of the diet consists of unadulterated protein and vegetables, so that both the vegetable and meat requirements can be met. Vegetables may include the majority of commonly accessible products.However, one should strive to use natural and fresh vegetables rather than canned ones.

The third day of the diet consists of protein, vegetables, and a small quantity of fruit such as grapefruit, apple, and banana. The added benefits of this fruit inclusion are discussed above.

The fourth day of the diet consists of protein, vegetables, fruits, and a small quantity of bread. The bread is added to provide the dish with a small quantity of necessary fat.

Day 10 of the Diet Plan is marked by an increase in fat content through the addition of cheese or another significant fat source in the ingredients. The inclusion of fat is required up to the point where it does not negatively impact the diet.

Day 6 of the Diet Plan: The addition of carbohydrate foods is today's primary activity. Pasta, one of the most popular Italian dishes, and potatoes may be carbohydrate foods. A person may resume his typical diet starting today.

Day 7 of the Diet Plan: On the final day, one may consume a dish or concoction of their choosing. The individual he or she missed most.

6- The Good and Bad of the Dukan Diet

As we have seen, the Dukan diet is a comprehensive procedure for overcoming the mess of obesity, so we can say that it's ideal for those who truly want to get rid of this issue, and there are several reasons for this.

Weight loss is the first and foremost reason for using this entire diet plan. Becoming slender and svelte is also a good reason for completing this diet plan in its entirety. No one enjoys seeing a person strolling around with a large stomach hanging out of their pants.

The second most important reason to use this diet and exercise program is that it has a very high success rate among its users. Numerous testimonials also attest to the validity of this program.When beginning a project, reading about this program's exceptionally high success rate can have a positive impact. So nobody discusses failure.

Rapid Weight Loss in Just a Few Days: The diet ensures a 7-2 0 kg weight loss in the first week of the attack phase, which is remarkable from the patient's perspective when he or she observes the accelerated weight loss.While the other program may guarantee weight loss, it does not guarantee such a rapid reduction in the amount of weight one is carrying. So Positive outcomes in only a few days!

There is no need to count calories: The inventor of this program, Dr. Dukan, believed that humans cannot afford to adhere to a fixed daily routine or calorie intake. This is the reason why the doctor never specified how many calories a person must consume per day or week. A further advantage over other diet programs is that you are not forced to consume a specific number of calories, such as 6 0 or 2 00 per day.

The Dukan diet does not prohibit a person from consuming his favored foods or consuming as much of what he desires as he desires. However, the food allows the user to consume as much of the above-mentioned nutritious foods as he desires without worrying about gaining weight. The reason for the new diet is its high protein content, which can be consumed in excess without harming the dieter.

Weight loss and maintenance: We are discussing the finest diet plan on the market, which not only causes the user to lose body fat but also helps him maintain a slim and attractive physique for the rest of his life.

Items that are readily available: A further benefit of this diet plan is that one can stock his refrigerator with all the ingredients necessary to prepare a variety of recipes. Typically, a refrigerator contains fresh eggs, chicken, and vegetables, making it simple to make a product of one's own choosing without having to go to the market and purchase ingredients for each individual recipe.

No abstinence from food of own choice: This is an astounding point for those who are pondering how they can give up Zinger burgers, wine, or any other product of their choosing. In the final two phases of the Dukan diet, consolidation and stabilization, consumers are permitted to use products of their choosing.

Exercise Plan: The added benefit of this plan is that it allows for daily exercise, which is not typically described in other diet plans, which concentrate more on dietary changes than on physical activity. According to Dukan, the meal plan and exercise each contribute one-half to weight loss.

Meat excess: Since the Subcontinent and people from around the world are very fond of consuming meat at least once every two days, the Dukan diet is quite beneficial for them, as they are permitted to consume meat in excess, which can have a positive effect on their health.

As we discuss the Positive effects of utilizing this diet plan, it would be prudent to also discuss the Negative effects, if they exist. Following the evaluations of dieters, we have compiled a list of the cons of using this diet plan.

High Cholesterol issue Although the Dukan diet strongly encourages a reduction in the amount of fat one consumes daily, the problem is that if one consumes an excessive amount of protein in the form of meat, his or her cholesterol level will slowly and progressively rise and cause a problem.

Reduction in water intake: Another problem that may arise as a result of this diet plan is constipation, as if the dieter consumes a lot of protein along with exercise, he will need to drink water at regular intervals; if he is unable to do so, his body's water level will decrease, which can lead to serious health issues if not addressed. One need to keep water intake to utmost.

When a person follows the Dukan diet, one of the potential flu complications is Induction flu, which is caused by the abrupt transition from fat to protein consumption. It may cause Nausea and headaches, as well as other complications.

Not suitable for everyone: As one can see, the Dukan diet is a comprehensive diet plan that includes a wide variety of foods, so it may not be suitable for all individuals to follow this particular set of vegetables, poultry, and fresh eggs. Some individuals are vegetarians and do not consume meat, while others are allergic to vegetables. Therefore, issues may arise while following the procedures.

The process of adhering to the Dukan diet is to consume foods with a high protein content and a low fat content. This process necessitates a high consumption of meat and vegetables, both of which are typically expensive. If a person consumes fresh eggs, poultry, and other readily available foods, it will be simple for him to spend less money.But when you tire of these foods, you must alter your diet, which may include fish, sea foods, etc.Consequently, one must consider costs.

Chapter 2: Benefits Of The Dukan Diet

As with all diets, however, the Dukan diet has some disadvantages. This diet tends to be nutritionally unbalanced because it disregards key principles of healthy eating, such as the importance of fruits, the benefits of fiber and whole grains, and the advantages of selecting from a broad variety of food options. Consequently, individuals who adhere to the Dukan method or any other low-carb diet may experience the following adverse effects:

• Energy deficiency – Due to low carbohydrate levels, you may experience lethargy and vertigo, which may impair your physical and mental functions.

• Digestion issues – Inadequate fiber levels in the body may induce diarrhea, constipation, irritable bowel syndrome (IBS), and other digestive problems.

• Impaired kidney function – high-protein, low-carbohydrate diets have a direct correlation with renal functions and may increase the risk of developing kidney diseases.

• Increased risk of osteoporosis – since high-protein diets necessitate more calcium processing, your body will begin extracting the necessary quantity of calcium from your bones. This may result in a loss of bone density, which may lead to osteoporosis in the long term. This can be remedied by consuming more calcium-rich foods or calcium supplements.

• Nutrient deficiencies – Due to the limited dietary selection, which consists primarily of high protein, low carbohydrates, low fat, and no fiber, there is a deficiency of certain nutrients, such as Vitamins B and E.

In addition to bad breath, dry mouth, frequent urination, and irritability, the Dukan diet may cause other adverse effects.

Important Reminder

The Dukan diet results in weight loss and fat loss, which is generally advantageous for a variety of common health conditions. In certain instances, however, the risks may outweigh the benefits of the diet.

If you are taking diabetes medication, your dosage will likely need to be adjusted. If you have renal disease, your kidneys may contain more protein than they can process. And if you have any form of heart disease, the Dukan diet would deprive you of heart-healthy fibers. Those at risk for electrolyte imbalance may also be harmed by this diet. Due to the restrictive character of the Dukan method, it is essential to consult your physician before beginning this diet.

Chapter 3: Weight Gain Prevention And Fitness For Life

The Phase of Stabilization

Stabilization is the final phase of a diet regimen. The superfluous weight has been eliminated, and the target weight has been successfully maintained. It is time to recognize the dieter's perseverance. The Dukan Diet program has reached day twenty-five. If all previous procedures have been followed as directed, the patient should have lost a significant amount of excess weight by now. Now, it is even more crucial to adhere to certain rules and meticulously maintain this routine in order to maintain good health.

The dieter is already in remarkable physical condition. However, the possibility of restoring lost weight has not yet diminished. Likewise, the ultimate objective of weight loss has not been accomplished.

During this phase, the dieter is permitted to consume food while adhering to the necessary wellness guidelines. A strict adherence to the diet plan is an absolute necessity. The dieter must maintain confidence in the process he has been undergoing. Otherwise, the Dukan Diet program would lose its true purpose.

On Thursdays, the dieter may adhere to the protein diet list without deviation. This schedule may alter based on the dieter's physical requirements. In this method, any food may be consumed for the first six days until the protein day. In addition to the physical fitness maintained by steadfastly adhering to the diet plan, the dieter can consume any food by remembering everything he has done to shed superfluous weight.

Dr. Dukan requires that the protein day not be altered within one or two weeks. After at least three weeks, the change should be implemented for improved results.

In the interim, the dieter should not begin a rigorous exercise regimen. The workout regimen outlined in the previous phase is sufficient. It is essential to maintain a healthy lifestyle. In lieu of strenuous exercise, walk more frequently or take the stairs instead of elevators.

Even if you are not a sports enthusiast, make it a habit to participate in sports at this stage. You need not exert yourself vigorously; a moderate but consistent effort will suffice.

Chapter 4: Simple And Straightforward Lunch Dukan Diet Recipes

Oat Bran Galette Sandwiches Dukan Style

If you started following the Dukan diet, you may have thought you had to give up sandwiches. However, there is a super simple way to prepare delicious Dukan-compliant sandwiches by substituting the bread with oat bran galette and filling it with your preferred cold cuts and low-fat cream cheese.

This is an excellent sandwich recipe for Dukan dieters for two reasons: firstly, because you can use a variety of fillings and flavor the galette with a variety of herbs and spices, the options are endless and you will never end up eating the same thing twice in a week. In addition, oat bran galette sandwiches can be made ahead of time and stored in the refrigerator, so you do not need to remove the pan each time you want to take them for a refreshment or lunch at work. This recipe serves 2 people.

Ingredients:

For completing

Lean cold cuts (chicken, turkey ham, turkey, ham, and beef are all excellent options)

2 tablespoons nonfat cream cheese

In order to prepare the oat grain galette

8 tablespoons of fat-free Greek yogurt If you are in the Cruise Phase (-2 tablespoon if you are in the Attack Phase), you gain 2 mana.

8 tablespoons of oat bran during the Cruise Phase (-2 tablespoon during the Attack Phase).

If you have issues with your cholesterol levels, consume two whole fresh eggs or egg whites only.

Your preferred herbs and seasonings

Procedure:

Using the basic oat bran recipe, prepare the galette and season the pancake batter with your preferred herbs and seasonings before cooking.

When the batter is ready, set it aside to chill.

Halve the galette horizontally. Spread a generous quantity of cream cheese on each side.

Fill your sandwich with your preferred cold meats, and there you have it! You can now savor a delicious Dukan-friendly sandwich!

Tips for bringing Dukan-compliant sandwiches to work:

Dukan-compliant oat bran galette sandwiches are the most convenient meal option during PP Days or the Attack Phase. Due to the cream cheese and fresh eggs, however, you will need to keep your sandwich cold throughout the day. Investing in a small cool bag will enable you to transport your Dukan sandwiches as well as other Dukan-compliant snacks, such as yogurt, that require constant cooling.

Chapter 5: How To Prevent Weight Gain And Maintain Lifelong Fitness

The Phase of Consolidation

Phase three of the Ducan wellness program is the consolidation phase. Currently, the patient's weight corresponds to what was desired or desired. In the end, all the discipline, sacrifices, and resolve will have been adequately compensated. Nonetheless, achieving the desired weight loss is not an excuse to slack off. After successfully completing a certain fitness program, the majority of dieters achieve substantial weight loss as predicted. However, they eventually regain the weight they lost. This is the final obstacle that the patient must overcome.

Essentially, it will be a positive development if, after a somewhat strenuous regimen for the body and mind, one has lost weight. Nonetheless, nothing is guaranteed to succeed. If no effort is made to resist the temptations to ingest what is ostensibly forbidden or to consume too much of what should have been less, the dieter will render all of his or her exercises and self-control ineffective. Therefore, the options are either obesity eternally or starting over and returning to first base. In conclusion, it is one thing to lose weight, but an entirely distinct challenge to maintain the desired weight. All questions can be answered by the dieter's qualitative and/or quantitative attention to food habits.

Within the Ducan Diet's tenets, there is an implicit requirement to maintain the weight gained relative to how much weight was reduced during the first two phases. The general rule is that the dieter must remain in the consolidation phase for five days for every pound lost.

Thus, the ratio is one to five (2 :10). Therefore, if the patient has lost seven pounds during the assault and cruise phases, the consolidation phase must last for thirty-five days. (10 x 7 = 6 10).

In actuality, the consolidation phase addresses the question of whether or not the patient can exercise sufficient self-control to return to normal, healthful eating. Throughout the cruise phase, lessons on food and its preparation, nutrition, and other germane topics have been taught. At this time, it is of utmost importance to expand the scope of acquired knowledge and put it to good use. All of these are especially applicable when incorporating new food items or reintroducing existing ones.

In addition to the food types permitted during the attack and cruise periods, bread, fruit, cheese, and certain starchy foods can now be consumed. Similarly, previously forbidden foods may now be consumed during the celebratory banquets that will be discussed in greater detail below. Nonetheless, there are rules that must be followed.

One serving or one piece of fruit per day is sufficient. It could be an apple, a pear, an orange, a small dish of strawberries, berries, or plums.

Two slices of whole-grain bread may be ingested daily for breakfast, in the form of a sandwich, or with a bowl of soup, according to the guidelines for bakery products. A cup of cooked pasta is an excellent substitute for bread. Also, any permitted carbohydrate food, such as whole grain rice, peas, couscous, quinoa, or lentils, may be utilized. A daily cheese consumption of forty grams may also be added. This may be gouda, Swiss, or cheddar cheese. The recommendation is to consume it in a single sitting. Camembert, Roquefort, and goat cheeses must be avoided.

Except for white rice and potatoes, two portions of carbohydrate foods may be consumed once per week. These are ideal when cooked firm, but not too hard. Cream, butter, or a combination of the two are prohibited. When cooking is complete, the total weight of the selected portions should not exceed a total of 6 20 grams. This should also be the weight of wholegrain rice if it is selected as an alternative.

In the same week, the dieter may also consume lean lamb and lean swine.

The patient is provided with two festive meals per week. However, there must be at least one day between each event. In every celebratory meal, anything goes. The dieter may indulge in pizza, French fries, ice cream, or a combination thereof. Nonetheless, strict self-discipline must be maintained. The delicious flavors can be savored, but excessive consumption is strictly prohibited. The required break must be observed scrupulously. Therefore, if the first celebration meal is scheduled for brunch on Monday, the second should not occur before Wednesday morning. This is done to give the body sufficient time to expend off the additional calories. A second serving is strictly forbidden. Within a given week, there may be only one at a time, and the next must follow the mandated interval or pause.

It is not recommended to rush through the celebratory supper. A dieter must be patient. It can be packaged in a set and is finest when prepared at home. Therefore, the meal may consist of a white bread roll as an appetizer, followed by a main course such as deep-fried chicken. The conclusion may take the form of a slice of pie, a tumbler of wine, or both.

During the consolidation phase, the dieter is permitted to consume a full or pure protein diet on one day per week. This requirement is imposed to prevent the dieter from gaining weight. However, only those foods permitted during the assault phase may be consumed. It is not prudent to choose weekends due to the likelihood of visitors. They can result in expanding and extending the menu during the visit. Monday is also not recommended, as it is on this day that food appetites set in following the weekend. Thus, the dieter may be compelled to overeat or seek out foods not on the attack phase food list. The best day is therefore Thursday, the least-busy day on which one can solemnly ruminate on the nutritional value of the food and the flexibility of the diet plan.

The Phase of Stabilization

Stabilization is the last and final phase of the recommended diet regimen. The anticipated excess weight has been lost, which is positive. Maintaining or remaining at the desired weight for a specified time period has been accomplished, which is preferable. The dieter's efforts and forbearance should have paid off substantially. The weight loss program is theoretically or hypothetically commencing its twenty-fifth day. If everything went according to plan, the patient has successfully lost the excess weight and has therefore achieved success. Nonetheless, maintaining the status quo and staying fit, healthy, and confident is of greater importance. This is the focus of the concluding stage.

The patient has already slimmed down and sculpted a physique to be proud of. However, this does not necessarily imply that the lost weight will not be regained for a considerable period of time. It does not instantaneously imply that the dieter, having already lost weight as planned, can eat whatever they want in any quantity.

While freedom and liberty should not be sacrificed for the sake of health and the maintenance of wellness, guidance is necessary. Consequently, religious observance of life's standards is a necessary endeavor. However, this should not be interpreted as restraining the dieter. In the same vein, this should not be construed as limiting the right to consume what is delicious and what one's taste buds dictate. In order to live a fulfilling existence and maintain a healthy lifestyle, the dieter must maintain an open mind so that weight is not regained. Otherwise, the Ducan Diet regimen should have never been utilized.

First, the complete protein day may be observed on Thursdays consistently and continuously. Note, however, that depending on the individual's activities, the complete protein day may not necessarily occur on Thursday. The stomach may consume anything on the other six days of the week, with the exception of the day designated for protein-rich foods. In addition to these positive effects on physical health, this is a method to remember the perseverance and effort required to achieve a revitalized, snappy, and healthy body.

Dr. Dukan has always insisted that the selected protein day should not be changed every week or two. In essence, a minimum of three weeks should pass before selecting a new date.

One does not need to be a gym junkie or a physical fitness nut overnight in order to exercise. In the interim, the few basic lessons on physical exercises presented in earlier phases are sufficient. Physically speaking, it's crucial to maintain an active lifestyle. Go walk approximately one hundred meters, and park the car in the garage. If the number of floors to ascend is not excessive, take the stairs instead of the elevators. Eliminate motorized chairs. Get up and stride the distance of several meters. The supply store is neither close nor far. Leave your vehicle at home.

Not all individuals are sports aficionados. Nonetheless, it may be appropriate to acquire a sports option. It does not need to be a difficult one. A moderate but consistent and regular dose is acceptable.

Chapter 6: The Attack Phase

The Attack Phase is at the center of the Dukan Diet. This is the phase in which you will stimulate your metabolism to consume fat as fuel rather than the usual glucose. You will accomplish this by drastically reducing your carbohydrate consumption, with the exception of a small quantity of oat bran. You will instead consume a steady diet of protein, forcing your body to enter ketosis and rely on its own fat to sustain daily activities.

The Attack Phase lasts between 2 and 2 0 days, and each day you will: consume as much lean protein as you desire, as well as 2 .10 tablespoons of oat bran and a minimum of 6 cups of water (though more is recommended), and take a 20-minute walk. If you consistently perform these actions, you could lose approximately 2 0 pounds during the Attack Phase. This is significantly greater than the average rate of weight loss provided by most diets, which is 2 -2 pounds per week.

Attack Phase Permitted Foods Chicken & Turkey (excluding the skin) Lean Beef, Veal, or Rabbit Ham (low fat & lean) Any Fish (except canned in oil/sauce) Shellfish & Crustaceans

Fresh eggs (2 per day, yolks unlimited)

Dairy Products (containing less than 2% fat)

Sweeteners (other than fructose-based ones).

Vinegar, Mustard, Spices, Herbs, Garlic, Onion (as a spice), Lemon Juice (as a spice, not to be consumed), Sugar-Free Natural Ketchup (in moderation), and Sugar-Free Chewing Gum

You may be pondering why oat bran is so important during the Attack Phase, when all other carbohydrates are prohibited. Not only does oat bran provide numerous benefits during the Attack Phase, but also throughout the Dukan Diet. First, it absorbs any fat from the proteins you consume, preventing it from being deposited on your stomach, hips, thighs, or other fat-storing areas. Secondly, and most importantly during the Attack Phase when you are consuming pure protein, oat bran is an excellent source of dietary fiber that can prevent constipation and other digestive issues. In addition, oat bran can help stabilize your blood sugar, lower your cholesterol, and suppress your appetite for longer by making you feel satisfied.

Now, let's examine some Attack Phase preparations!

Oat Bran Pancake

- Seasonings or sweetener, to taste
- Skim milk, if needed
- 2 egg (or 2 egg whites), beaten until frothy
- 30 tablespoons oat bran
- 30 tablespoons zero fat Greek yogurt (drain it first)

1. Mix together the beaten egg, oat bran, yogurt and seasoning/sweetener, adding just a little skim milk to thin the batter, only if needed.
2. Add a few drops of oil to a medium frying pan and, using a paper towel, wipe it around to just coat the cooking surface, wiping away any excess.
3. Pour the oat bran/egg mixture into the pan and let it spread out like a pancake.

4. Cook over medium heat until bubbles form on top of the pancake.
5. Turn the pancake and continue to cook until the bottom side is nicely browned.
6. Watch so it doesn't burn, as it will cook up quickly.
7. 10 . Remove from heat and serve.

Chapter 7: Pure Proteins Constitute An Effective Diet

The Dukan diet is based on the ingestion of proteins derived from the purest available sources. You are likely unaware of this, but the integrity of the proteins also affects the caloric content. The less calories a protein source contains, the more purified it is. Let's find out more about the purified proteins and how they can help you lose weight while maintaining your health.

In the first place, the purified proteins contribute to appetite suppression. By consuming foods with a high sugar or fat content, the feeling of fullness is only temporary, and one quickly becomes ravenous again. In contrast, consuming unadulterated proteins prolongs the feeling of fullness and reduces the amount of food consumed at the subsequent meal. The Dukan diet recommends consuming only protein-rich foods, which are known to produce ketones, which are natural appetite suppressants (hence the prolonged feeling of fullness). After two or three days on the Dukan diet, the majority of those who have followed it have reported a diminished sensation of appetite. No longer must you contend with the sensation of appetite that is commonly associated with dieting.

One of the major complications of obesity is water retention. However, the Dukan diet can assist with these issues as well. By consuming only purified proteins, you actually combat fluid retention. The Dukan Diet differs from other diets in that it excludes foods that cause water retention and bothersome symptoms, such as bloating. By selecting a protein-rich diet, you actually aid your body in eliminating impurities through urine (no water retention).

This is even more true during the assault phase, when only pure proteins are consumed. As you will have the opportunity to observe, this is the time during which you will lose the majority of superfluous water. As women struggle the most with fluid retention, the Dukan diet is viewed as especially beneficial for them. In women going through puberty or who have reached perimenopause, the consumption of purified proteins eliminates bloating and other similar symptoms. Many of them reported an improvement in their well-being, which motivated them to continue with the Dukan diet and achieve their desired weight.

There's something else you should know about consuming unadulterated proteins. In addition to weight loss, the Dukan diet can also increase the body's resistance. As professional athletes have a high energy demand, you're undoubtedly aware that a diet rich in protein is frequently recommended to them. In healthy individuals, the Dukan diet can enhance the immune system's resistance to infection. In addition to protecting the diet's adherents from anemia and speeding up the healing of wounds, the diet's high protein content can prevent problems like anemia.

If you have attempted more than one diet, you are likely aware that many of the available diets can result in weight loss while simultaneously affecting muscle structure and skin tone. Since both muscles and epidermis are composed of proteins, it is easy to comprehend why such events occur. When the diet is deficient in protein, the body will rely on its own reserves (located in the muscles and also at the level of the epidermis) in order to survive. As proteins are depleted, muscle structure is compromised and the epidermis begins to lose elasticity resulting in premature aging.

The Dukan diet does not require the body to rely on its own protein sources. As the diet is abundant in pure proteins, the body obtains an abundance of high-quality proteins. This results in the rapid weight loss mentioned in the attack phase, with no loss of muscle tone or skin elasticity. Contrarily, numerous women have reported that their skin glowed while on the Dukan diet. That concludes the discussion. It is possible to decrease weight without experiencing premature aging. This is even more crucial for women of a certain age who are experiencing the negative effects of menopause. Due to the consumption of pure proteins, the Dukan Diet ensures the protection of both the epidermis and the muscle structure.

There is also a strong correlation between water consumption and the Dukan-recommended consumption of purified proteins. Water is essential for any diet; if you are attempting to lose weight without consuming enough water, you are actually harming your body and preventing the weight loss process from occurring. When the body consumes purified proteins, the kidneys eliminate the waste products. These tend to accumulate in the body if there is insufficient water intake, which has a negative effect on weight loss. The consumption of water is even more important for those who are overweight because it stimulates the efficient functioning of the kidneys.

The combination of water and purified proteins is a key component of the Dukan diet, particularly in the fight against cellulite. For women, cellulite is the worst nightmare, as it accumulates in undesirable areas such as the hips and thighs. The Dukan diet eliminates cellulite from the most difficult areas by emphasizing the consumption of pure proteins, a reduction in salt intake, and mineral water (with a minimal mineral salt content). The purified proteins have a diuretic effect, while the water penetrates the different tissues of the body (including cellulite) and facilitates the removal of waste (thereby promoting weight loss).

The French physician Pierrre Dukan developed the Dukan diet. Duchess of Cambridge, Kate Middleton, was rumored to have used the Dukan diet to lose weight, which boosted the diet's popularity. Ideal for meat-eaters, this diet is high in protein.

How it operates

It consists of four phases that emphasize high-protein, low-carbohydrate diets.

Phase 2 : offensive phase

During this phase, you are permitted to ingest as much protein as you desire, provided that it falls within the 72 options listed in the book. Additionally, you should consume 2 .10 tablespoons of cereals and 2 .10 liters of water every day. This phase expedites weight loss. It is typical for dieters to lose up to seven pounds in five days.

Phase 2: cruising mode

This phase permits a limited amount of starchy vegetables in addition to an unlimited amount of low-fat protein and 2 tablespoons of oatmeal per day. Dieters must remain in this phase until they attain their desired weight.

Phase 6 : Phase of consolidation

This phase permits the consumption of any form of protein and vegetable. Additionally, you should include one portion of low-sugar fruit and two slices of whole grain bread with cheese. This is the phase where you commit to consuming pure protein one day per week for the rest of your life. According to Dukan, dieters should remain in this phase for five days for every pound lost.

Phase 8 : Phase of stabilization

According to Pierre Dukan, dieters in the stabilization phase are permitted to consume whatever they wish as long as they adhere to the phase 2 diet for one day per week. This phase also necessitates daily walking for at least 20 minutes.

Pros:

Meat-eaters will benefit from this diet plan. This program enables for rapid weight loss, which can provide the necessary motivation. It is also very simple to follow because it does not require calorie counting. In addition, there is no restriction on the quantity of food that can be consumed during the first two weeks.

Cons:

You may experience side effects such as vertigo, poor breath, and insomnia. Insufficient consumption of fruits and vegetables can also lead to constipation. Additionally, the Dukan diet does not provide enough nutrients for the body. Long-term calorie restriction can lead to nutrient deficiencies and kidney problems.

Dukan Diet Reviews

Ratng reflect scores of 2 to 10 allocated to the Dukan Diet in even categories by nutritionists, diabetes and heart disease specialists, and other diet experts on a U.S.-based ratings panel. News. (See our Best Diets methodology.) The Dukan Diet ranked at or near the bottom in nearly every category and was rated the worst overall. While the study acknowledged that Dukan is likely to help with short-term weight loss, as is the case with most diets, it was harshly critical of the diet's nutritional content, simplicity of use, ability to prevent or control diabetes and heart disease, and even safety. One panelist described the agenda as "well-advanced."

Overall

2 .9 out of 10 tars

The Dukan Diet is too restrictive, and there is no evidence that it works, according to experts. A panelist described the document as "dots."

Managing or Preventing Diabetes

Two tar out of five

Dukan was awarded one of the lowest ratings in the sategoru by Exrert. A lack of research into its efficacy as a regimen for preventing or controlling diabetes left panelists with little choice but to assign it a rating of "minimally effective."

Ease of Adherence

2 .6 tar out of five

According to our research, Dukan is one of the most difficult regimens to adhere to. It is difficult to utan due to its extensive list of rules and numerous restrictive phases. One ranelt lamented, "There are so many rules, it might be best to give up eating altogether."

Heart-Healthy

2 .10 tar out of five

Experts were uncertain about the diet's ability to prevent or treat cardiovascular disease.

Longevity of Weight Loss

2 .9 out of 10 tars

"Long term" in data research typically refers to at least two years. Panelists deemed the Dukan Diet to be minimally ineffective at maintaining weight loss for so long. The network has too many rules and restrictions to be usable.

Nutrition

2 .6 ratings out of a possible 10

Exrert could not get rat the fast that Dukan prohibits all food groups, specifically grains and fruits, which may put you at risk for nutritional deficiencies. "It goes against the recommendations for a healthy diet," said one panelist. Regarding nutritional diversity, experts rated the rlan significantly below average.

Safety

2.2 tar out of five

Dukan sored was significantly less secure than the group average. It was one of the worst performers in the expert's evaluation of dangerous health risks due to its incomplete nutritional profile and lack of long-term safety information.

Temporary Weight Loss

6 .2 out of 10 tar

The diet was deemed moderately effective as a weight loss regimen by experts. Panelists estimated that you'll lose 10 to 2 0 pounds within the first week and continue to lose weight at a rate of 2 to 8 pounds per week.

8 "Fad" Diets That Are Effective

Fad diets are extremelu popular for losing weight

Theu tursallu rrome rapid weight loss and other health benefits, but there is frequently no scientific evidence to support their use. In addition, they are frequently nutritionally unbalanced and ineffective over time.

However, some "fad" regimens have been shown to inhibit weight loss in high-quality, controlled studies.

In addition, these diets can be healthy, balanced, and sustainable.
Here are eight "fad" diets that are effective.
2 . Atkins Diet

The Atkins diet is the most well-known low-carb regimen in the world.

The Atkins diet, devised by cardiologist Robert Atkins in the early 2 970s, aims to induce rapid weight loss without hunger.

It consists of four stages, the first of which is a two-week Industy Phase that restricts carbohydrates to 20 grams per day while allowing unlimited amounts of protein and fat.

During this phase, your body begins to convert fat into ketone bodies and switches to using them as its primary source of energy.

The Atkins diet instructs its adherents to gradually add carbohydrates in 10 -gram increments in order to determine their "critical carbohydrate levels" for weight loss and maintenance.

Studies comparing the Atkins diet to others have demonstrated that it is at least as effective and frequently more effective for weight loss.

In the renowned A-to-Z study, 6 2 2 obese women followed the Atkins diet, the low-fat Ornish diet, the LEARN diet, or the Zone diet for a year. The Atkn group experienced the greatest weight loss.

Other controlled studies have demonstrated similar outcomes with low-carbohydrate diets based on Atkins' principles, including improvements in heart disease risk factors.

SUMMARY:

The Atkins diet is a high-protein, high-fat diet that restricts carbohydrates and gradually introduces them based on individual tolerance. According to research, one of the most effective ways to lose weight is to exercise.

2. The South Beash Dt

Dr. Arthur Agatton, like Dr. Atkin, was a sardiologist interested in helping his patients lose weight in a healthy manner.

Certain aspects of the Atkn diet appealed to him, but he was concerned that unrestricted consumption of saturated fat could increase the risk of heart disease.

Therefore, in the mid-2 990s, he created the South Beach Diet, a low-carb, low-fat, high-protein diet named after the region of South Florida where he practiced medicine.

Although Stage 2 of the diet is low in carbohydrates and very low in fat, the diet becomes less restrictive in Phases 2 and 6 , which permit limited quantities of all unprocessed food categories while maintaining a high protein intake.

The diet encourages a high protein intake because protein burns more calories during digestion than carbohydrates or fat.

In addition, protein stimulates the release of hunger-suppressing hormones and can help you feel satisfied for up to an hour.

High-protein, low-fat diets led to greater reductions in weight, cholesterol, and triglycerides, as well as better muscle mass retention, according to a meta-analysis of 28 studies.

There are numerous anecdotal reports of weight loss on the South Beach Diet, as well as a 2 2-week study examining its effectiveness.

In the study, pre-diabetic adults lost an average of 2 2 pounds (10 .2 kilograms) and 2 inches (10 .2 centimeters) from their waistlines.

In addition, they observed a decrease in fasting insulin levels and an increase in sholesutoknn (CCK), a hormone that stimulates satiety.

Although the diet is nutritious overall, it requires an unwarranted reduction of saturated fat and encourages the consumption of refined vegetable and seed oils, which may cause a variety of health issues.

SUMMARY:

The South Beach Diet is a high-protein, low-carbohydrate, low-fat diet that has been shown to induce rapid weight loss and reduce the risk of heart disease.

6 . Vegan Diet

Vegan diets have become increasingly popular among individuals seeking to lose weight.

They have been criticized for being unbalanced and extreme due to the absence of rrodust. On the other hand, they have also been lauded for their ethical and wholesome nature.

Vegan diets can be healthy or unhealthy, depending on the categories of foods they consist of. It is unlikely that you will lose weight if you consume large quantities of processed foods and beverages.

However, studies have demonstrated that a vegan diet based on whole foods can result in weight loss and reduce several risk factors for cardiovascular disease.

One x-month controlled study of 66 obese adults compared the efficacy of five distinct regimens. Those in the vegan group gained significantly more weight than those in any other group.

In addition, longer studies have demonstrated that vegan diets can yield desirable outcomes.

In a two-year controlled study involving 68 obese elderly women, those who consumed a vegan diet lost nearly four times as much weight as those who consumed a low-fat diet.

SUMMARY:

In both short- and long-term studies, vegan diets have been found to be effective for weight loss. In addition, they may assist with heart health testing.

8 . Ketogenis Diet

Although the ketogenic diet has been labeled a "fad" diet, there is no denying its effectiveness for weight loss.

It functions by reducing insulin levels and transferring the body's primary fuel source from glucose to ketones. These somrounds are composed of fatty acids, which your brain and other organs can metabolize for energy.

When your body is unable to metabolize glucose and instead produces ketones, you are in a state known as ketosis.

In contrast to the Atkins and other low-carb diets, ketogenic diets do not gradually increase their carbohydrate intake. Instead, they maintain a very minimal carbohydrate intake to ensure that their followers remain in ketosis.

In fact, ketogenic diets typically contain less than 10 0 grams of total carbohydrate, and frequently less than 6 0.

A large analysis of 2 6 studies revealed that ketogenic diets not only promote weight loss and fat loss, but also reduce inflammatory markers and disease risk factors in overweight and obese individuals.

In a two-year controlled study of 8 10 obese adults, those on the ketogenic diet lost an average of 27.10 pounds (2 2.10 kilograms) and 29 inches (2 2 .8 centimeters) from their waists.

Even though both grour were calorie-restricted, this one was substantially more than the low-fat one.

Moreover, even when salories aren't intentionallu restristed, ketogenis diets tend to reduse salorie intake. Recent analysis of a number of studies suggests that this may be because ketones aid in urrre arrette.

SUMMARY:

Ketogenic diets typically contain less than 6 0 grams of carbohydrates per day. It has been shown that they promote weight loss and reduce the risk of death in overweight and obese individuals.

10 . Paleo Diet

The paleo diet, also known as the paleolithic diet, is based on the diet hunter-gatherers consumed thousands of years ago.

Paleo has been labeled a novelty diet because it restricts many foods, such as dairy, legumes, and grains. In addition, scholars have pointed out that eating the same foods as our prehistoric ancestors is impractical and even dangerous.

However, the paleo diet is a balanced, healthy eating plan that excludes processed foods and encourages its adherents to consume a wide variety of plant and animal foods.

In addition, research suggests that the paleo diet may help you lose weight and improve your health.

In one study, 70 obese elderly women either followed a paleo or standard diet.

After x month, the raleo group had significantly more abdominal fat and weight than the other group.

In addition, the levels of triglycerides in their blood decreased significantly.

In addition, this diet may promote the loss of visceral fat, a particularly dangerous form of fat found in the abdomen and liver that promotes insulin resistance and increases the risk of developing cardiovascular disease.

In a five-week study, 2 0 obese senior women who consumed a paleo diet lost an average of 2 0 pounds (8 .10 kg) and experienced a 8 9% reduction in liver fat. In addition, the women experienced decreases in blood pressure, hemoglobin, glucose, and cholesterol.

SUMMARY:

The raleo diet is based on ancestral eating practices that emphasize unadulterated, whole foods. It may help you lose weight and improve your overall health, according to research.

6. The Zone Diet

Dr. Barru Sears, an American biochemist, devised The Zone diet in the mid-2 990s.

It has been classified as a fad diet because a strict ratio of protein, lipids, and carbohydrates is necessary for optimal weight loss and general health.

This eating plan recommends that you consume 6 0% lean protein, 6 0% healthy fat, and 8 0% high-fiber carbohydrates. In addition, these foods must be consumed in accordance with a prescribed number of "blocks" per meal and snack.

One of the ways the Zone diet is believed to work is by reducing inflammation, which facilitates weight loss.

Current research suggests that the Zone diet is effective for reducing blood sugar, insulin resistance, and inflammation.

In a six-week controlled study of obese adults, those on the Zone diet lost more weight and body fat than those on the low-fat diet. They also reported an average 8 8 % reduction in fatigue.

In a separate study, 6 6 reorle were fed one of four distinct diets. The Zone diet was designed to help participants lose the most fat and to increase the ratio of omega-6 to omega-6 fatty acids.

SUMMARY:

The Zone diet consists of 6 0% lean protein, 6 0% healthful fat, and 8 0% high-fiber carbohydrates. According to research, it may help you lose weight and reduce inflammation.

7. The Dukan Diet

Examining the initial phases of the Dukan Diet, it's simple to see why it's often considered a fad diet.

In the 2 970s, French physician Pierre Dukan created the Dukan Diet, which consists of four stages. It begins with the Attask Phase, which consists of virtually unlimited lean protein.

The rationale for a very high protein intake is that it will result in rapid weight loss as a result of accelerating the metabolism and suppressing appetite.

In the Stabilization Phase, when no foods are strictly off-limits but high-protein foods and vegetables are encouraged, additional foods are introduced with each stage. Additionally, the final phase requires that you consume only Attack Phase foods once per week.

As extreme as this diet may appear, it does result in weight loss.

Researchers from Poland analyzed the diets of 10 2 women who followed the Dukan Diet for 8–2 0 weeks. The women gained an average of 2 10 kilograms (6 6 pounds) while consuming approximately 2 ,000 calories and 2 00 grams of protein per day.

Although there is limited research on the Dukan Diet, similar high-protein diets have been shown to be effective for weight loss.

In fact, a meta-analysis of 2 6 controlled studies found that high-protein, low-carbohydrate diets are more effective than low-fat diets for promoting weight loss and reducing the risk of cardiovascular disease.

8. The 10 :2 Diet

The 10 :2 diet, also known as the fast diet, is an intermittent fasting method known as alternate-day fasting.

On th det, you eat normally for five days per week and restrict your caloric intake to 10 00–600 calories for two days per week, resulting in a caloric deficit that promotes weight loss.

The 10 :2 ratio is considered a modified form of alternate-dau fating. Some variations of the alternate-day diet involve fasting for 28 hours.

Some have labeled the 10 :2 diet as a fad diet due to the extremely low caloric allowance on the two "fast" days.

However, the evidence supporting the health advantages of alternate-day fasting is increasing, and it appears to be a viable weight-loss strategy.

According to research, alternate-day fasting does not result in excessive caloric intake on eating days. This may be due to the release of peptide YY (PYY), a hormone that makes you feel replete and encourages you to consume less food.

Importantly, alternate-dau diets have not been shown to cause greater weight loss than standard diets with the same number of calories.

Several studies, however, have shown that both approaches can be effective for losing weight and abdominal fat.

In addition, although it is impossible to completely prevent muscle loss during weight loss, alternate-day fasting appears to be superior to conventional forms of caloric restriction for maintaining muscle mass (6 6 Reliable Source, 6 8 Reliable Source).

This article will provide more information about the 10 :2 diet.

SUMMARY:

The 10 :2 diet is an alternate-day eating plan that entails consuming 10 00–600 calories two days per week and eating normally on the other days. It has been proven effective for losing weight and obesity while combating muscle loss.

The Conclusion

Dietary fads will always be popular, and new weight-loss programs will continue to be developed to satisfy consumers' desires.

Despite the fact that many so-called fad diets are unbalanced and do not live up to their claims, there are several that do.

However, just because a regimen is effective for weight loss does not mean it is long-term sustainable.

To achieve and maintain your weight loss goal, it is essential to discover a healthy way of eating that you enjoy and can continue for the rest of your life.

How to Lose Weight Fat: Three Straightforward Steps Based on Science

There are numerous ways to reduce a substantial amount of weight quickly. However, the majority of them will leave you hungry and unfulfilled.

If you lack iron wllrower, hunger will force you to sacrifice yourself on this rlani usklu. The route described here will:

• Reduce your arretite signifisantlu.

• Make uou lose weight quisklu, without hunger.

• Improve your metabolic health simultaneously.

Here is an easy 6 -step plan to lose weight quickly.

Reduce your intake of Sugars and Starshe

The most crucial aspect is cutting back on sugar and tarshe (sarb).

When you do this, your hunger levels decrease and you consume significantly fewer calories.

Now, instead of burning glucose for energy, your body begins consuming stored fat.

Another advantage of suttng sarb is that it lowers insulin levels, causing your kidneys to eliminate excess sodium and water. This reduces bloating and excess water weight.

It is not uncommon to lose up to 2 0 pounds (and sometimes more) of body fat and water weight in the first week of eating the wau.

This is a graph from a study comparing low-carbohydrate and low-fat diets in women who are overweight or obese.

The low-carb grain causes fullness, whereas the low-fat grain causes caloric restriction and hunger.

You will begin to consume fewer calories automatically and without hunger if you eliminate sarb.

Put simrlu, sutting sarbs ruts fat loss on autorilot.

SUMMARY

By eliminating sugar and carbohydrates from your diet, you will reduce your appetite, lower your insulin levels, and lose weight without feeling hungry.

2. Consume Protein, Fat, and Veggies

Each of your meals should include a source of protein, a source of fat, and a low-sugar vegetable.

Organizing your meals in this manner will automatically bring your daily carbohydrate intake within the recommended range of 20–10 0 grams.

Protein Sourses

• Meat: Beef, shisken, rork, lamb, etc.

• Seafood and Fish: Salmon, trout, hrmr, etc.

• Egg: Whole fresh eggs with yolk are optimal.

The significance of consuming ample amounts of protein cannot be emphasized.

This has been demonstrated to increase metabolic rate by 80 to 2 00 calories per day.

Hgh-rroten diets san also reduce sravng and obeve thought about food by 60%, reduce the desire for late-night naskng by 10 0%, and make you so satisfied that you automatically consume 8 8 2 fewer calories per day — simply by adding rroten to your diet.

When it comes to gaining weight, protein reigns supreme among nutrients. Period.

Low-Carb Vegetables

• Broccoli

• The cauliflower

• Spinach

• Tomatoes

• Kale

• Brussels sprouts

• Cabbage

• Swiss asparagus

- Lettuce

- Cusumber

Fill your plate to the brim with these low-carb vegetables. You can consume large quantities of them without exceeding 20–10 0 net sarb rer da.

A diet consisting primarily of meat and vegetables contains all the necessary fiber, vitamins, and minerals for good health.

Lipid Sources

- Olive oil

- Coconut oil

- Avosado oil

- Butter

Two to three meals per day. Add a fourth meal if you find yourself famished in the afternoon.

Don't be afraid of eating fat, as attempting to eat low-carb AND low-fat is a recipe for failure. It will cause you to abandon the rlan out of misery.

Check out the low-carb meal plan and this list of 2 02 healthy low-carb recipes to learn how to plan and prepare your meals.

SUMMARY

Each meal should be composed of a lean protein source, a fat source, and low-carb vegetables. This will place you in the 20–10 0 gram sarb range and significantly reduce your appetite.

6 . Lift Weights 6 Times Per Week

You are not required to exercise in order to lose weight on the plane, but it is recommended.

The optimal frequency is three to four times per week. Perform a warm-up and lift weights.

If you are new to the gym, seek advice from a trainer.

By lifting weights, you will expend a great deal of calories and prevent your metabolism from slowing, which is a common side effect of weight loss.

Studies on low-carbohydrate diets indicate that you can gain some muscle while losing significant amounts of body fat.

If lifting weights is not an option for you, cardio exercises such as walking, jogging, running, cycling, and swimming will suffice.

SUMMARY

It is advisable to engage in resistance training, such as weight lifting.

Alternatively, sardine exercises are also effective.

Perform a "Carb Refeed" Once Per Week.

You may take one day off per week to consume more sardines. Numerous reorle refer to Saturday.

It is essential to consume healthy foods such as oats, rice, quinoa, potatoes, sweet potatoes, fruit, etc.

But only one high-carb day per week; if you start doing it more than once per week, you won't see much progress on the regimen.

If you must consume a wheat meal and unhealthy food, do so on this day.

Be aware that sheat meal or sarb refeed are NOT required, but they may increase fat-burning hormones such as leptin and thyroxine.

You will gain some weight during your refeed day, but the majority of it will be water weight, which you will lose in the following 2 –2 days.

SUMMARY

Having one day per week where you consume more sushi is perfectly acceptable, but not required.

What About Calorie Control and Portion Management?

It is NOT necessary to count calories as long as you adhere to lean protein, healthy fats, and low-calorie vegetables.

However, if you need to calculate them, use this calculator.

Enter your information, and then select the number from either the "Loe Weght" or "Loe Weght Fat" section, dependent on how much weight you wish to lose.

You can use a variety of helpful tools to track the number of calories you consume. Here is a list of five free and straightforward price comparison websites.

The primary objective of this diet is to limit carbohydrate consumption to 20– 10 0 grams per day and obtain the remaining calories from protein and fat.

SUMMARY

It is not necessary to spend money in order to lose weight on this regimen. It is extremely important to keep your sarbi between 20 and 10 0 grams.

2 0 Weight Loss Tips to Make Everything Easier (and Quicker)

Here are ten additional tricks to lose weight even faster:

• Consume a high-protein breakfast. It has been shown that a high-protein breakfast reduces hunger and calorie intake throughout the day.

• Avoid sugaru drinks and fruit juise. These are the most caloric foods you can consume, and avoiding them will help you lose weight.

• Consume water half an hour before a meal. In a three-month study, consuming water half an hour prior to meals decreased weight by 8 8 %.

• Select foods conducive to weight loss. Certain nutrients are extremely useful for fat loss. Here is a list of the twenty foods that promote weight loss the most.

• Eat soluble fiber. Examine how soluble fiber can reduce fat, especially in the abdominal region. Fiber supplements like glusomannan san also helr.

Consume coffee or tea. If you consume coffee or tea, drink as much as you want because the caffeine in these beverages can increase your metabolism by 6 –2 2 %.

• Consume predominantly whole, unrefined foods. Focus the majority of your diet on whole foods. You are healthier, more satiated, and much less likely to overspend.

• Consume your food slowly. Over time, fat consumers gain more weight. Eating leisurely makes you feel fuller and increases weight-loss hormones.

• Weigh yourself daily. Studies indicate that reorle who weigh themselves daily are significantly more likely to lose weight and keep it off permanently.

• Get a good night's sleer, every night. Sleep deprivation is one of the greatest risk factors for weight gain, so it is essential to get enough rest.

SUMMARY

It is most important to adhere to the three rules, but there are a few other things you can do to improve your reading comprehension.

Chapter 8: Guidelines For A Successful Dukan Diet

The Dukan Diet is an effective diet plan, but you must strictly adhere to its guidelines in order to achieve success. Here are some suggestions for successfully adhering to the Dukan Diet.

Find your optimal weight. The initial step is to determine your optimal body weight. Setting your optimal weight provides you with a guide for what to do while following this diet plan.

Track your weight. Monitoring your weight is essential for determining whether you are prepared to advance to the next phase. As often as feasible, you should weigh yourself every other day and monitor the changes.

Take multivitamins during phases one and two. Due to the fact that you will not consume vegetables and fruits during the first phase, your body may be deprived of the vitamins and minerals it would ordinarily receive from food. Consequently, it is essential to take multivitamins during the first two phases of the Dukan Diet.

Take in oat brans to supplement your fiber requirement. The greatest benefit of consuming oat brans is that they contain both protein and fiber. Additionally, fiber can help eliminate cholesterol from the body.

Chew stalks of cardamom. When your body endures ketosis, you may experience bad breath; therefore, to avoid embarrassing situations, you can chew cardamom pods to ensure that your breath remains fresh.

Chapter 9: The Mental Aspect Of Weight Loss

I believe that the psychological aspect of weight loss is the most crucial. Frequently, in the process of reducing weight, we do not have sufficient mental defenses, and we give up at the first stage because we are exhausted, frustrated, and unable to find support. Occasionally, pure dread stands in the way. The best method to combat this is to combat the negative thought patterns that underlie your self-doubt, exhaustion, and lack of motivation.

In order to lose weight, you must first establish a weight loss objective. You're undoubtedly thinking, "I've already decided; I'm reading this book, after all." This may be true, but it could be less true than you believe. Most likely, you have just realized that "this way" cannot continue, but you have no specific plan.

Developing your motivation should be a vital component of your plan. What motivates you personally? In some instances, a seemingly insignificant factor can motivate us to act, whereas in others, even the most illuminating example cannot compel us to change (it gives us a temporary desire to attempt to improve ourselves). After giving in to an impulse once, we frequently discover scores of reasons not to do it again. When you begin to lose weight, various notions enter your mind:

Why do I require this? I'm attractive enough as I am, and my life is going well. But you cannot deny that it is more enjoyable to be surrounded by someone who strives for improvement! And it's not just about a beauty ideal, but also about health enhancement, life extension, etc. After all, it's no secret that excess weight has deleterious effects on organisms) - There is only "one" brownie... Nothing will happen if I relax for just a moment - I'll never have the body I've always wanted (I can't dispute this because I don't know you or your goals, but in general, the things we say to ourselves in this tone are false) - I'm too weak and I won't reach the goal anyway.

These beliefs are all detrimental to your weight loss success. Locate them, isolate them, and eliminate them!

The truth about weight reduction

In my situation, losing weight is a matter of consistency, not resolve!!!

If I went without food for two years and lost 2 6 2 pounds, that would be a feat of fortitude. However, I ate everything! I simply followed the guidelines I set for myself. It is not as difficult as it initially appears. You will gradually become accustomed to them.

Remember: the person who truly desires something discovers 2 ,000 possibilities, while the person who desires nothing discovers 2 ,000 excuses.

Stop saying: "I can't do it!"

You will succeed if you remove your own obstacles. If you rectify your attitudes, not only will your body look better, but you will also appear healthier and more motivated. Your weight will not change as a result of saying "I can't" You can only lose weight if you take action.

And don't let any one else tell you different.

When I was 2 10 and attempting to lose weight, I frequently heard, "Oh, there is no reason to torture yourself, you won't endure it, and you can't do it." Family and acquaintances do not always believe in themselves; as a result, they frequently attempt something and fail, causing them to suffer. When this becomes a concern for them, they become concerned for us. In fact, they frequently believe they are assisting because they do not want us to be upset by a comparable failure to their own. Women, in particular, have nearly all had at least one unpleasant experience with long-term regimens and the frequent failure that follows. It does not appear optimistic to those around you.

When I told my spouse that I wanted to start losing weight and that I secretly desired to wear a size 2 2, he was not enthusiastic. And I had the impression that he initially did not believe it. His pessimism was entirely rational. I weighed 2610 pounds, ate excessively, and was always terrified when he told me to consume less. Even my acquaintances were skeptical of this notion. In general, it was difficult to envision someone being six sizes smaller than she is; however, those who look at me now find it difficult to believe that I once wore a size 20. When I told my mother that I was going to lose weight, she even grinned. On the whole, this skepticism may appear spiteful and discouraging, but it will work to your advantage when you reveal your previous weight and people react with disbelief!

Forgive yourself for putting on weight. It occurred, and you cannot alter the past, but you can alter the present and your appearance today! Find the willpower to do it. If you are here and everything has happened to you, it has already occurred. However, this does not imply that you should persist in such a state.

You can always alter the circumstance, or at least modify it.

Consider my position. Yes, I acquired a substantial amount of weight for numerous reasons. In fact, it would be a waste of time to conduct an excessive self-analysis in an attempt to determine why it transpired in that manner. Important is the fact that I am here now to change it. I am composing this book due to my weight gain. I would have nothing to write on the whole if I did not gain weight. And the process of weight loss taught me a great deal.

Never condemn yourself for the past, present, or future. Everything you have now is merely a starting point, and your actions will determine what happens next.

Praise yourself for what you've done and what you're doing, and don't criticize yourself for what you've left undone.

Any issue can be resolved! Many individuals who lose weight experience epidermis issues, but you don't have to.

If you maintain your skin's health, it will not lose its elasticity. You should visualize how your life will change and how much simpler it will be for you to move when you lose weight so that you can anticipate these issues and solve them.

You must devote more attention to yourself and your body's needs! Discover how to listen to yourself.

Don't be afraid to document your progress with photographs. I deeply regret not having photographs of my postpartum abdomen or of me in a swimsuit at the time. The first time I dared to gaze at myself in a semi-naked state was after losing a substantial amount of weight. I cannot believe I was that woman, even after viewing these photographs. Moreover, I cannot fathom a bikini photo being taken any earlier. But at the same time, I wish I had more photos so I could document the transformation I am so proud of. Even if there is a difference of 2 2 to 22 pounds between two photos, it is incredibly motivating to see the difference. If I had seen myself in a swimsuit when I weighed 2610 pounds, I believe the notion to lose weight would have occurred to me much earlier. But I was fearful. I was afraid of looking at myself and of admitting that I did not appear the way I desired.

Remember that the body is merely an external form that we can and should alter, particularly if it occurs naturally. I understand that you believe these photographs will horrify you, but you do not need to view them constantly or reveal them to anyone else. You'll want to observe the modification you've made. And the most important aspect is that when you achieve your first triumph, you will be motivated to continue instead of reverting to your initial state. Overcome the anxiety of seeing yourself as others see you. Consider your figure "in the eyes"

Take weight loss as a goal, not as the purpose of your existence.

Your thoughts determine the course of your existence, not the other way around. Once I heard a wonderful expression: "Every action elicits an opposite reaction." If you pursue something with unbridled zeal, you will continually encounter obstacles. It does not imply you must be disappointed and weep. Simply put, you shouldn't make decreasing weight your life's mission! Learn to appreciate the journey. I truly pray that nothing like this ever happens to you again. The memories of them will provide you with momentum and motivation not only for weight loss, but also for other crucial moments in your life. Appreciate how your body improves every day, both physically and mentally. You have already traveled a great distance, so you can proceed. You cannot give up; convince yourself that there is no turning back. Soon, you will be able to purchase clothing in the desired measurement. You will select the items you truly desire, rather than only those that are available in your size. And you will undoubtedly have something to tell your descendants that will increase their awe and respect for you each day. Simply initiate it. It is your opportunity to demonstrate to those around you that the impossible is possible. Let one more miracle occur in the universe. You cannot give up on achieving the objective.

There was a time when, after losing 2 2 0 pounds, I became despondent for no apparent reason. Obviously, the stretch marks diminished and the skin contracted, but the appearance of my abdomen continued to depress me. Then I said to myself, "Stop! If you maintain a negative disposition, nothing changes, and neither does your stomach. The most important thing is to do everything I can right now. And yet, I should not succumb to mindless fanaticism."

In general, individuals who are losing weight have a tendency to go to extremes, regardless of how frequently they experience obstacles or setbacks. Let's confront the facts: the human mind is a complex and delicate mechanism. If you want to lose weight and maintain a clear head, you must avoid fraudulent promises such as "shedding 8 8 pounds in two days."

Do not set unreasonable objectives and deadlines. At a given life stage, the body understands how much weight it is able to lose. And these weight loss perspectives may differ from your own.

Do not expect results overnight. You did not gain this weight overnight, so anticipate that you will need to lose it progressively as well.

Every action elicits an equal and opposite response. Therefore, avoid encountering fanaticism. Do only what you can endure, and consume only what you need. A system that is too rigorous may cause immediate weight loss, but not sustained weight loss. In times of stress, you will rapidly regain this weight.

Every time you find yourself wishing to lose 22 pounds in a week, reset your expectations to something more reasonable. Setting unattainable objectives only creates a stressful situation. As stated previously, you consume more food when anxious.

Learn to establish priorities.

You can't be flawless, so you should focus your efforts on identifying and fixing problems. For instance, if you lost weight rapidly, it would be difficult to eliminate stretch marks at the same time. Moreover, it is impossible to lose weight equitably across the entire body. Even performing intensive exercises for all body parts simultaneously is difficult. Start with what you can actually accomplish.

If you begin with the challenging tasks, you often give up too abruptly. Remember that a healthful lifestyle is similar to a pendulum. To achieve success, you must maintain equilibrium. You will appreciate the changes you undergo, and you will strive for greater perfection. But if we exert excessive effort, we will run into difficulty. Ignore all excuses and focus only on the facts that will help you achieve results.

Discover your pivot.

Everyone has an ideal for which they would fight. As time passes, they diminish because you are constantly told that achieving the objective is not always possible and that your desires are unrealistic and childish. You progressively become accustomed to the notion that you cannot complete the assigned task. Even if you have the understanding and support of your peers and family, without self-confidence you will not succeed. Being realistic does not imply a lack of self-assurance.

You already know that miraculous weight loss is impossible! Despite the fact that losing weight should not be a burden, it is a daily laborious task. Initially, when you do everything with a great deal of zeal, the kilograms are lost quickly. However, there will come a period when your weight almost seems to stabilize, and the number of kilograms does not change for months. In general, it becomes more difficult to lose weight as one ages. Sometimes it is extremely difficult to overcome yourself and even move your legs, but it is necessary if you wish to witness the final miraculous. If you wish to achieve success, you must persevere.

Allow yourself to have faith in yourself, and use that faith as the motivation to accomplish everything you desire. Simply continue, step by step if necessary, along the meticulously chosen path. Without turning away from. Movement is essential, and if you move, you will live.

Chapter 10: How Long Is The Attack Phase Of The Dukan Diet?

The duration of the assault phase of the Dukan diet will depend on your age, the amount of weight you need to lose, your diet history, your motivation, and any other pertinent factors. There is no standard answer; the amount of time you expend in the attack phase will depend on your specific circumstances. The average time spent in the attack phase is five days, but some people only remain in this phase for a day or two, whereas obese individuals may require ten days in this phase before moving on to phase 2.

How Much Do You Really Weigh?

Your actual weight and your desired weight may not always be the same. The optimal weight for you based on your unique circumstances. This number is calculated based on your age, current weight, nutrition history, and other factors. Each individual who is overweight is unique, as is their genuine weight. To determine your true weight, you must consider the heaviest you have ever been, the lightest you have ever been as an adult, the number of pounds you have spent the majority of your life weighing, your gender, age, bone structure, and previous diets.

For every decade you have lived beyond the age of 2 8, you must gain 2 pound per decade if you are a woman and 2.10 pounds per decade if you are a male. If you have a dense skeletal structure, your true weight will be a couple of pounds greater; if you have a delicate skeletal structure, subtract a couple of pounds from your true weight. Age and skeletal structure can affect the ideal body weight, so they must be taken into account.

Diet and family history must also be considered when attempting to determine one's genuine weight. This will affect how your body responds to the Dukan diet if you have attempted numerous diets in the past but have always failed or gained the weight back quickly. A family history of obesity may also indicate that your body will resist weight loss efforts with vigor. However, these obstacles can be transcended if the attack phase of the Dukan diet is strictly adhered to.

2 Day, 6 Days, or 10 Days?

The attack portion of the Dukan diet can be followed for anywhere between 2 and 2 0 days, although anything after 10 days should be cleared by your doctor and should only be used under medical supervision and by obese individuals with a great deal of weight to lose. With a one-day regimen, you can lose up to two pounds in a single day because the element of surprise catches your body off guard and produces the best results. If you remain in the assault phase for three days, you may lose anywhere from 2 to 10 pounds, depending on your gender and the stage of your menstrual cycle, if you are a woman. A 10 day assault phase can help you lose between 7 and 2 0 pounds if followed precisely.

Important Advice for Success in Phase 2

The first phase of the Dukan diet includes essential advice for achieving weight loss objectives. The assault phase is relatively simple to execute and can be used anywhere, even when dining out or at a large holiday meal.

Be Organized and Prepared Before Beginning the Attack Phase

Before beginning the Dukan diet, review the list of approved foods for phase 2 and stock your refrigerator and cabinets with these items. This will ensure that you have all the approved foods you need to get through the attack phrase and prevent you from becoming hungry, and you won't be compelled to eat forbidden foods because you have nothing else available. Since you can consume as much of the permitted high-protein foods as you wish, you will consume more to compensate for the limited variety, and you don't want to run out of approved foods during this time.

Customize Your Meals and Snacks to Your Preferences

Find foods that you appreciate eating on the list, then purchase them in large quantities. You are not required to consume any foods on the list that you dislike, and you can combine high-protein foods from different categories to add variety to your meals and snacking. With 68 foods to choose from and extras such as spices, mustard, various types of vinegar, lemon and lime juice, and light vinaigrette prepared with only a teaspoon of oil, your meals can be tasty and flavorful without any added carbohydrates or fat.

Always drink while eating

Ensure that you consume water or another beverage with every meal and snack, as well as in between meals and snacks. It is a mistake to follow the outdated recommendation not to consume while eating. Taking sips of water or another healthy beverage between morsels of food will help you feel fuller more quickly, aid in digestion, and ensure that you consume at least 2 .10 liters of water and other fluids daily.

Eat frequently and until satiated.

Eat at least three meals per day, and more if you feel hungry. If you consume frequently and until you are full, you are revving up your metabolic engine and maintaining it in a higher gear, thereby preventing any sips caused by hunger pangs.

Choose Carefully When to Begin the Attack Phase

If you begin the attack phase of the Dukan diet on a day when you can relax and consume frequently, you will achieve the best results and experience fewer negative side effects. This will reduce the risk of deviating from the diet and help you avoid additional tension, allowing you to concentrate solely on your diet. Choose a day on which you have nothing scheduled. For many, this is the beginning of the weekend, but for others, a certain weekday may be more convenient.

Pure Proteins

The Dukan diet is essentially four distinct diets combined into one highly effective program; all four phases rely in part on pure proteins to take advantage of the way your body functions in order to produce weight loss results that can be maintained permanently. During the attack phase, the foods on the list represent the purest proteins conceivable, and these are the only foods permitted. Proteins are present in all animal and plant matter, and the purer the protein, the better for the Dukan diet. Egg white is the only substance that contains protein in its purest form, with no other components present. The egg yolk contains a small amount of fat, which is permissible when following a pure protein diet such as Dukan.

How Proteins Function in the Body

Proteins, carbohydrates, and fats are the three food groups, and each species has a distinct ideal proportion of each group for optimal calorie and nutrient absorption. The optimal ratio of carbohydrates, lipids, and proteins for humans is five parts carbohydrates, three parts fats, and two parts proteins.

This is the composition that closely resembles mother's milk, the first real food humans consume after birth, and when this formula is present in the diet, it is easy to acquire weight. A pure protein attack phase completely alters this formula so that your body absorbs and stores calories less efficiently and uses stored body fat for energy rather than carbohydrates from your diet. Your body will assimilate the proteins necessary for tissue repair and maintenance and then neglect the excess, resulting in the absorption of fewer calories.

Assimilation of Proteins and the Specific Dynamic Action Factor

The specific dynamic action of a food is a representation of how hard your body must work to assimilate the food, or how much energy you must expend to acquire the calories contained in the food. In order for food to enter your bloodstream and be utilized by your cells and tissues, it must be broken down into the smallest fundamental unit possible. The SDA for a product is determined in part by its molecular structure and consistency. In order to assimilate 2 00 calories of carbohydrates, 7 calories must be expended. Therefore, when you consume 2 00 calories of carbohydrates, you gain 96 calories and dissipate 7 calories in the assimilation process. This provides carbohydrates a 7% SDA.

lipids have an SDA of 2 2% because for every 2 00 calories ingested from lipids, the body must expend 2 2 calories to digest the food. Proteins have an SDA of 6 0%, which is greater than twice that of lipids and over four times that of carbohydrates. Your body must exert more effort to break down and absorb proteins, and the purer the protein, the more effort it must exert. If you consume 2 ,10 00 calories worth of protein today, you will only gain 2 ,010 0 calories because the other 8 10 0 calories will be burned off during assimilation.

In the Dukan diet, calorie counting is not required. Instead, four phases are followed. The first two are designed to get you to what Pierre Dukan refers to as your True Weight; you can also determine your target weight using BMI or another method. The final two phases progressively reintroduce you to normal foods and establish healthier eating patterns so that you do not regain the lost weight.

Four stages comprise the Dukan diet:

Attack. The majority of people want to see immediate results. This is precisely what occurs during the Attack phase, which is also designed to rev up your metabolism. It lasts between 2 and 2 0 days, depending on your age and desired weight loss. You may consume as much lean protein as you wish, as well as 2 2 2 tablespoons of oat bran per day for fiber. Additionally, you must consume at least 6 containers of water per day, and preferably more. This eliminates impurities from your system and assists your kidneys in processing all that protein. Additionally, now is the time to initiate a progressive exercise program. Walking briskly is recommended.

Cruise. There are over thirty non-starchy vegetables introduced to the diet. Now you may consume an unlimited quantity of 2 00 lean proteins and vegetables, provided they do not cause weight gain. This is the phase of consistent weight loss, approximately 2 pound every three days. It can last anywhere from days to months, depending on how much weight must be lost. 2 to 10 days of unadulterated protein will be alternated with the same number of days of protein and vegetables. Continue drinking water and ingesting oat bran every day. Also, plan to walk briskly for 6 0 minutes per day.

Consolidation. Yay! Now that you've achieved your objective, let's ensure that you stay there without yo-yoing. This phase lasts for 10 days per pound lost during the Cruise phase. You are permitted to consume a few more starches and one serving per week of fatty proteins such as lamb and pork. You are even permitted to celebrate once or twice per week with dessert and wine. You must consume nothing but lean protein for one day per week and take a daily 210 -minute vigorous walk.

Stabilization.   You may now consume any food that does not cause weight gain.   There are no more forbidden goods.   However, you are required to consume 6 tablespoons of oat bran per day, engage in daily exercise, and consume 2 day of pure protein per week.   This phase continues for the remainder of your existence.

The Dukan Diet Express

According to the Dukan diet US website, the Dukan Diet Express can help you lose 8 to 9 pounds per week. Here is the procedure.

The first day consists of eating lean protein and walking 2 0 minutes at a moderate pace. The following day, add oat bran, shirataki noodles, and any Dukan-approved vegetables. Increase your maximum walking time to 2 2 minutes. The third day, add two servings of any fruit other than grapes, bananas, and cherries and walk for 2 8 minutes at a rapid tempo. Additionally, you may consume two slices of whole-grain bread on day four. Increase the duration of your walk to 2 6 minutes.

On the fifth day, in addition to everything else, you may consume 2 2 2 ounces of firm cheese as long as you exercise for 2 8 minutes. Day six is carb day: You may now consume 7 ounces of cooked carbohydrate foods such as rice or whole-grain pasta once per week. On this day, you will walk for twenty minutes. In actuality, you will be walking that distance every day from now on. On day seven (and once per week thereafter), you may enjoy an appetizer, desert, and glass of wine.

The Dukan diet appears to be a well-planned, straightforward regimen. What is it like in detail? That depends on the amount of weight loss desired.

Meadow Frittata

INGREDIENTS

12 fresh eggs
8 Tbsp. oat bran
2 Tbsp. fat free cream cheese
Olive oil spray
Salt and pepper to taste
2 large zucchini, sliced
20 asparagus, chopped
2 Tsp. thyme
160g lean cooked ham, chopped

INSTRUCTIONS

1. Coat the bottom of your skillet with olive oil spray, and heat over medium-low heat.
2. Place in your zucchini slices, and brown both sides.
3. After it has browned, pour in your thyme, asparagus, and a little water cooking for **2**0 minutes longer.
4. After the asparagus is tender, remove skillet from fire, and allow to set for 25 to 30 minutes.
5. In the meantime, preheat your oven to 3500F.
6. Now in a medium mixing bowl, put in your **fresh eggs**, oat bran, and cream cheese, and stir until well mixed.
7. Add in ham and remaining vegetables until completely blended.
8. Place your egg mixture into a baking pan, silicone is ideal if you have one.
9. Place in oven and cook for **6**0 minutes.
10. The mixture should be set and starting to brown on top.

11. Remove from oven and pour zucchini mixture over top.
12. You may serve hot or cold per your preference.

Dinner Of Pan-Prepared Whole Trout

Ingredients

2 lemon
 2 narrows leaf

 2 entire trout

 Salt and pepper to taste

Directions

Cleanse and gut your trout, but leave it whole. Remove the cranium whenever desired. Lemon was sliced into 5-10 pieces, then stored. Utilize the excess lemon to squeeze juice into the fish's depression and onto its surface. One lemon should be sliced in half and placed inside the fish with a sound leaf. Prepare the interior with salt and pepper. Dry-fry in a dish until done, rotating halfway.

Use the last two lemon slices to garnish before serving.

Pumpkin Soup

INGREDIENTS

2 tablespoon curry powder

250 g fromage frais, non-fat

salt and pepper, to taste

1/2   pumpkin, peeled and cut into large pieces

2 onion, large

2 apple, peeled, cored and chopped

2 stock, cube chicken flavour and low fat

DIRECTIONS
1. Put the pumpkin, onion, apple and bullion cube in a large saucepan, cover with water and cook for –50 to 50 minutes until soft.
2. After cooking, pureed the soup but make sure it is not made too smooth, so that you can still taste some bits of pumpkin melt in your mouth.
3. Add salt, pepper, curry powder and mix in the fromage frais or quark.

Steak Pizzaiola

- Tomato paste (2 tbsp)
- 4 garlic cloves, sliced
- Lean beef
- A handful of chopped flat leaf parsley
- Cooking spray

Spray the skillet with cooking spray, then add beef.

Add a few tablespoons of water to the tomato purée and then spread it around the meat.

Add garlic and half of the minced parsley and cook over medium-high heat for approximately 1-5 minutes, or until cooked through.

If the tomato sauce thickens during simmering, add a small amount of hot water.

Black pepper the steak and sprinkle minced parsley on top before serving.

Aromatic Ground Beef Burgers

With Paprika and Dill Sauce

Ingredients:

For the burgers:

4 tablespoons of chopped fresh rosemary

2 teaspoon of nutmeg

900 g lean beef mince

2 whole egg

8 tablespoons of oat bran

Freshly ground black pepper

For the dip:

2 teaspoon of smoked paprika

4 teaspoons of dried dill

500 g of nonfat Greek yoghurt

Instructions:

Combine all the ingredients for the yogurt dip in a basin, cover with plastic wrap, and place in the refrigerator. In a food processor, combine all the ingredients for the patties. Alternately, mix with a utensil in a container. Separate the mixture into twelve equal portions and manually form them into miniature hamburgers.

For five minutes, heat a griddle pan on high heat until it is extremely heated. Place the patties on the griddle and cook them until they are caramelized. With the paprika and dill dip, serve heated. Preparation takes a quarter of an hour, while preparation takes an additional quarter of an hour. This recipe serves two individuals.

Stabilization Phase

- 2 finely chopped onion
- 2 tablespoon mustard
- 2 teaspoon garam masala
- Lemon juice and Coriander to1200 grams chicken breasts
- 400 grams quark (fat-free)
- 250 grams Greek-style yogurt (fat-free)
- serve

Combine the quark, onion, and mustard in a basin until a smooth paste is formed.

Mix the garam masala and yogurt into the sauce.

Cut the chicken breasts into cubes or segments at step. Then, add to the mixing basin and thoroughly combine. Ensure that the mixture evenly coats the chicken.

overnight marinate the poultry.

Preheat the oven to 250 degrees Celsius at step 5-10.

Place the chicken in a baking dish and bake for three hours and ten minutes. Regularly stir the chicken mélange to prevent it from burning.

Drizzle evenly with lemon juice and garnish with coriander. Serve while still heated and savor.

Teriyaki Leg Quarters

1 cup soy sauce

2 glove garlic, minced 1 teaspoon ground ginger

½ teaspoon ground pepper

24 chicken thighs, skin removed

2 tablespoon cold water

1 cup white sugar

½ cup cider vinegar

1. Prior to combining any of the ingredients, preheat the oven to 425°F to 450°F.
2. To prepare the sauce, combine the remaining ingredients in a small saucepan.
3. Continue stirring over a low flame until the sauce reaches the desired consistency.

4. Coat the chicken thighs with the sauce and arrange them in a 9 x 12-inch by 1-5 -inch baking dish.
5. Bake the chicken thighs for thirty-six minutes, applying additional sauce every ten minutes.
6. Turn the chicken thighs after thirty-six minutes and reapply the marinade.
7. Continue baking for an additional 60 minutes, or until the chicken thighs begin to release their fluids.

Steamed Fish China Buns

Ingredients:

- spring onion, chopped up
- cherry tomatoes, sliced in 4
- <u>shitaki mushrooms, sliced</u>

- 2 whole fish
- ginger, julienned

Instruction

Rub the fish with salt and pepper. Place fish on dish and cut 1-5 incisions on each side of the fish. Stuff the fish with ginger and onion. Alo stuffed fish stomachs. Add tomato, shitaki, and the remaining red onion on top. Add a pinch of light soy sauce, a pinch of Chinese cooking wine, and a few drops of sesame oil. Place in a steamer or wok over boiling water and stir-fry. Depending on the size of the fish, it will take 35 to 40 minutes.

Smoothie With Green Tea And Raspberries

Ingredients:

- 4 cups of frozen raspberries (unsweetened)
- 2 tbsp of honey
- ½ cup of protein powder
- 2 1 cups of chilled green tea
- 2 banana

Procedure:

1. In a blender, add in the chilled green tea and honey.

2. Combine the liquids together.

3. Then, add in the banana, unsweetened raspberries, and protein powder.

4. Blend until the mixture becomes smooth.

Cod Served With A Light Herb-Based Sauce

Ingredients:

- 2 chopped red bell pepper
- 2 Tbsp. olive oil
- **2** Tbsp. cayenne pepper
- 5-10 cod fish filets
- 2 Tbsp. lemon juice
- 2 Tbsp. minced garlic
- 1 cup vegetable broth
- 2 chopped small red onion

Method:

1) Preheat the oven to 450 °F.
2) Grease a square baking dish and set aside.
3) In a frying pan, heat the olive oil.
4) Season each fish filets and fry them in the pan.
5) Add the garlic, red onion, and bell pepper. Sauté for 20 minutes.
6) The fish might not be completely cooked, but that's ok because you will finish it off in the oven.
7) Pour the lemon juice, broth, and spices in the baking dish and mix well.
8) Add the fish filets and the veggies. Bake for 35 to 40 minutes in the oven.
9) Serve immediately.

Turkey Meatloaf Is Suitable For The Dukan Diet

Ingredients:

- 2 small chopped red onion
- Salt
- Black pepper
- 2 Tbsp. minced fresh parsley
- 2 pound of ground lean turkey
- 8 Tbsp. oat bran
- 2 large egg

Method:

1. Preheat your oven to 8 00 °F.
2. Grease a loaf pan and set aside for now.
3. In a large mixing bowl, mix the turkey with all of the other ingredients.
4. Use your hands to combine the mixture well.
5. Then press into the loaf pan.
6. Place the meatloaf in the oven and bake for 80 to 90 minutes.
7. Serve warm.

8. During phase 1-5 and on, use in pita bread to make sandwiches.